HOMOEOPATHY

An Introduction to the use of classical homoeopathic medicines in the treatment of common ailments and conditions

Recommended by
HOMOEOPATHIC DEVELOPMENT FOUNDATION LTD

CONTENTS

INTRODUCTION

There are many homoeopathic remedies available that can be used to treat most minor illnesses and conditions. The aim of this leaflet is to provide a basic explanation of how homoeopathy works so that it can be used safely for self care and first aid situations.

This book should not be viewed as a substitute for expert advice from a homoeopathic doctor. Further, where symptoms persist beyond a reasonable period you should always consult a qualified doctor. However, used as a handy reference, this book will aid in the treatment of everyday complaints.

The fact that homoeopathic remedies are without side effects and are safe even for small children makes them eminently suitable for self medication in the treatment of common complaints for all the family.

Today homoeopathy is practised by qualified doctors worldwide and over the years has become recognised as an effective and safe form of medical treatment. In the United Kingdom, homoeopathy is recognised by an Act of Parliament and all homoeopathic medicines are available on prescription under the National Health Service.

WHAT IS HOMOEOPATHY?

Homoeopathy is a natural and safe alternative to conventional medicine and is suitable for both adults and young children to use. In its most basic form, homoeopathy is the treatment of an illness with a substance which, when taken by a healthy person, would produce symptoms similar to those shown in the person who is ill.

Current medical practice takes the viewpoint that symptoms are a direct result of an illness and seeks to treat the ailment by suppressing the symptoms. Homoeopathy works in reverse to this. It views any symptom as the body's natural reaction to combat the illness and looks to stimulate rather than suppress the reaction.

Homoeopathy therefore, is essentially a natural healing process, providing remedies to assist the patient to regain positive health by stimulating the body's own natural forces of recovery. In its current form, homoeopathy is based on three principles which are:

1. A medicine that in large doses produces the symptoms of the disease will, in small doses, cure that disease.

2. By extreme dilution, the medicine's curative properties are enhanced and all the poisonous or undesirable side effects are lost.

3. Homoeopathic medicines are prescribed individually by the study of the whole person, according to basic temperament and responses.

HOW DID HOMOEOPATHY BEGIN?

The basic principle of homoeopathy 'like cures like' (simila similibus curentur) dates back to the fifth century. It was at this time that the Greek philosopher, Hippocrates actively started to believe that a patient's own powers of healing were vital in choosing an appropriate cure and should be encouraged. Hippocrates set about collecting hundreds of remedies to help prove this principle. Despite his commitment, his theory was largely ignored until the eighteenth century when homoeopathy was reborn.

Modern homoeopathy owes itself to Dr Samuel Hahnemann, a German physician who further developed the concept. Hahnemann was so appalled by the medical practices of his day that he was keen to find a method of healing that was safe, gentle and above all effective. Hahnemann, like Hippocrates, believed that humans have a capacity for

4

healing themselves, and that the symptoms of a disease represent the individual's struggle to overcome an illness. He reasoned that instead of suppressing symptoms one should seek to stimulate them and so encourage and assist the body's natural healing process.

Hahnemann became so discontent with the medical practices of his day that he left the medical profession and turned to translation to earn a living. It was when Hahnemann was translating 'A Treatise on Materia' by Dr Edward Cullen, that he came across the idea that was to be the beginning of a whole new philosophy of medicine. In his 'A Treatise on Materia' Cullen stated that quinine, a natural substance purified from the bark of the cinchona tree, was a good treatment for malaria. Hahnemann investigated the effects of quinine on himself and his friends and found that in a healthy person, quinine produced the same symptoms as malaria - fever, sweating, shivering, etc.

Hahnemann went on to discover that remedies obtained from animal, vegetable and mineral sources were equally effective. Over a long period of time, Hahnemann and his assistants took small doses of various substances and carefully noted down the symptoms that they produced. These were called 'provings' and Hahnemann built up a complete 'drug picture' for each substance depending on the feelings and symptoms that they caused in each of his volunteers.

Hahnemann's next step was to test his theory on ill people. Hahnemann questioned each of his patients in detail, asking them about their way of life, their attitudes and their general health and with this information managed to build up what he termed as a 'symptom picture'. He then prescribed each patient a substance whose 'drug picture' matched most closely to the patient's 'symptom picture'. Hahnemann discovered that the closer the match the more successful the treatment, therefore advocating his 'like cures like' theory - i.e. a remedy and a disease which produce the same symptoms cancel each other out in some way. He named this new principle of healing 'homoeopathy' from the Greek words homoeo meaning 'similar' and pathos meaning 'suffering'.

Hahnemann used many substances that were highly poisonous and to ensure their safety he gave them to his patients in small, dilute doses. He developed a three-step process whereby each substance was diluted, shaken and then banged on a hard surface in order to release the energy of the remedy – this process later became known as succussion. Hahneman tested these diluted remedies and found that the more times a remedy had been diluted and succussed the faster and more effectively it worked - i.e. although the remedies were theoretically weaker they were actually more potent. These were called 'potentizations' and in modern homoeopathy the term 'potency' is used to describe the dilution and strength of a remedy. The process of dilution formed the second principle of homoeopathy, which is that 'by extreme dilution, the medicine's curative properties are enhanced and all the poisonous or undesirable side effects are lost'.

During his research Hahnemann discovered that people varied in their responses to each remedy depending on their basic temperament. He found that patients suffering from the same disease often required different remedies, whilst there were groups of patients suffering from different diseases who all benefited from the same remedy. So, homoeopathy concentrates on treating the patient rather than the disease and this became the third principle of homoeopathy.

Dr Samuel Hahnemann is renowned as being the father of modern day homoeopathy and founded the three basic principles of homoeopathy:

1. A medicine that in large doses produces the symptoms of a disease will, in small doses cure that disease.

2. By extreme dilution, the medicine's curative properties are enhanced and all the poisonous or undesirable side effects are lost.

3 Homoeopathic medicines are prescribed individually by the study of the whole person, according to basic temperament and responses.

QUESTIONS AND ANSWERS

1. Is homoeopathy safe?

Homoeopathy is one of the safest forms of OTC medicine available because the active ingredients are present in extremely low concentrations. Homoeopathy is renowned as being safe, non toxic and non addictive and is prepared in laboratories licensed by the Department of Health to stringent standards of quality.

Homoeopathy, like many conventional tablets and pillules, has small amounts of lactose so patients who are lactose intolerant should take care when using these products. As with all conditions treated over the counter, patients should seek the help of their homoeopathic practitioner or doctor if their symptoms persist or deteriorate.

2. Is homoeopathy effective?

Since the early nineteenth century homoeopathy has proved effective for many millions of people worldwide and it has often been used successfully where other forms of medicine have failed. In more recent years medical journals have published positive reports of the results of scientific research into homoeopathy.

3. Is homoeopathy recognised officially?

Homoeopathy was recognised by an Act of Parliament in 1948, as a safe alternative form of medical treatment. Homoeopathy is practised by doctors who are fully qualified through conventional medical training and it is recognised by the General Medical Council. Homoeopathic prescriptions are available under the National Health Service.

4. What are homoeopathic potencies?

The potency is the number of times the mother tincture has been diluted. For example, if one drop of mother tincture is added to 99 drops of diluent (water or alcohol) and succussed (vigorously shaken) this is known as 1c potency. If one drop of this is then diluted in the same way, the resulting solution is 2c potency. This dilution can be repeated many times until the desired potency is achieved. The most commonly used potencies are 6c and 30c.

5. How do I know which potency to use?

The principles of homoeopathy mean that the more dilute a remedy, the more potent it becomes. As a general rule, for most acute and long-standing ailments, the 6c potency is most suitable. In emergencies and in many chronic conditions, 30c remedies are better. However, it is more important to select the correct remedy than to use the right potency.

6. What reactions can I expect on taking the treatment?

A slight increase in symptoms may be experienced at the start of treatment. These are known as 'aggravations' and are a sign that the body's own natural healing powers are starting to work. If this happens you should stop taking the remedies until the aggravation subsides and then restart. If the symptoms continue to worsen after stopping the remedy, it could be that the condition is worsening and you should seek advice from your GP or pharmacist.

7. What should I do if some symptoms improve but others don't or if new symptoms appear?

In this case, a second remedy should be started based on the remaining or new symptoms.

8. Does taking a larger dose have a greater effect?

No. It is the frequency of taking the dose that matters, not the number of tablets or pillules. Always follow the instructions on the pack regarding the dosage.

9. How should homoeopathic medicines be stored?

All homoeopathic medicines should be kept in their original container, away from direct light and strong smelling substances such as toothpaste, mint, perfume, aromatherapy oils, mothballs, menthol inhalants and rubefacients. If any tablets, pillules or granules are spilled they should not be returned to the container.

10. How should homoeopathic medicines be taken?

The recommended dosage should be followed, which varies according to product and potency. The remedies should not be taken with any food or drink or when the mouth is tainted by tobacco or any strongly flavoured food or toothpaste. The remedies should be tipped directly into the mouth without being handled and they should be sucked, chewed or allowed to dissolve in the mouth – do not swallow them whole.

11. Can more than one homoeopathic remedy be taken at once?

A classical homúopath would say that only one remedy should be taken at one time – monotherapy – and that this remedy should be sufficient to treat all of a patient's ailments. However, modern homoeopathy does not necessarily follow this rule. In some cases two or even three remedies are taken together to treat different symptoms. The disadvantage of this is that the patient may not know which of the remedies cured them.

12. Can homoeopathic medicines be taken with ordinary drugs?

It is safe to take homoeopathy whilst taking allopathic medicines. However, any side-effects that are caused by the allopathic drug may complicate the symptom picture and make the correct choice of a homoeopathic medicine more difficult. Always follow your doctor or homoeopath's advice.

13. Can homoeopathic medicines be taken while pregnant?

Although it is generally considered safe to take homoeopathic medicines whilst pregnant, they should only be taken on the advice of the patient's GP.

14. Are homoeopathic remedies safe for children?

Yes, even babies can take them safely. The remedy should be dissolved in a small amount of water or crushed between two spoons.

15. Can animals be treated with homoeopathy?

Homoeopathy is as effective for animals as it is for humans. There is an increasing number of veterinary surgeons practising homoeopathy in the United Kingdom. Addresses are available from the British Homoeopathic Association in London.

POPULAR HOMOEOPATHIC REMEDIES

There are several thousand homoeopathic remedies available in a wide range of different potencies of which the 6c and 30c potencies are the most common. The following is a list of homoeopathic remedies that are stocked in most pharmacies and health food stores. Remedies that have not been included in the list are generally available either by mail order or from specialist homoeopathic pharmacies.

1. Aconitum napellus (**Aconite**)

2. Apis mellifica (**Apis mel.**)

3. Argentum nitricum (**Argent. nit.**)

4. Arnica montana (**Arnica**)

5. Arsenicum album (**Arsen. alb.**)

6. Belladonna (**Belladonna**)

7. Bryonia alba (**Bryonia**)

8. Calcarea carbonica (**Calc. carb.**)

9. Calcarea fluorica (**Calc. fluor**)

10. Carbo vegetabilis (**Carbo veg.**)

11. Euphrasia officinalis (**Euphrasia**)

12. Gelsemium sempervirens (**Gelsemium**)

13. Graphites (**Graphites**)

14. Hepar sulphuris (**Hepar sulph.**)

15. Hypericum perforatum (**Hypericum**)

16. Ignata amara (**Ignatia**)

17. Ipecacuanha (**Ipecac.**)

18. Kalium bichromicum (**Kali bich.**)

19. Kalium phosphoricum (**Kali. phos.**)

20. Lycopodium clavatum (**Lycopodium**)

21. Mercurius solubilis (**Merc. sol.**)

22. Natrum solubilis (**Nat. mur.**)

23. Nux vomica (**Nux vom.**)

24. Pulsatilla nigricans (**Pulsatilla**)

25. Rhus toxicodendron (**Rhus tox.**)

26. Ruta graveolens (**Ruta grav.**)

27. Sepia (**Sepia**)

28. Silicea (**Silicea**)

29. Sulphur (**Sulphur**)

30. Thuja occidentalis (**Thuja**)

SELECTING AND USING THE CORRECT HOMOEOPATHIC REMEDY

This guide to self-treatment relates to common ailments and conditions that can be treated in the home environment. If you are suffering from a chronic condition, or where the symptoms are serious or prolonged you should always consult a doctor or a qualified homoeopath first.

Selecting the remedy

1. Note your main symptoms and any strong likes and dislikes that may arise from them.

2. Study the 'index of symptoms' (pages 14–26) to find the selection of remedies that can be used to treat individual symptoms.

3. Carefully look at the 'medicines and their indications' (pages 27–35) and select the medicine that most closely matches your symptoms.

4. When selecting a remedy you do not always have to experience all the symptoms listed nor do you have to exhibit all the likes and dislikes – these are often expressed as an extreme which may not always apply. Simply try to match up with the set of symptoms most similar to yours.

Selecting the potency

There are several thousand homoeopathic remedies available in a wide range of different potencies of which 6c and 30c are the most commonly found in the retail environment.

6c potency for most common or long standing ailments

30c potency for emergencies or chronic conditions.

Dosage and frequency

• Typically, 2 pillules every 2 hours for the first six doses.

• Thereafter, 2 pillules 4 times daily for up to five days or until the symptoms improve, or as directed by your doctor or homoeopath.

The first six doses give the body's own recuperative processes a suitable stimulus – thereafter, four times a day is adequate to maintain this effect.

Tablets may be crushed if being administered to a child. If symptoms worsen or persist always consult a doctor or homoeopathic practitioner. Pregnant women should always consult a doctor or practitioner before using homoeopathic remedies.

Response to a homoeopathic remedy

When taking a homoeopathic remedy sometimes the symptoms may become worse. Do not be alarmed as this indicates that the medicine is working. If this happens postpone the dose until this increase or 'aggravation' as it is known, has passed.

GENERAL PATIENT ADVICE

Antidoting

The minute quantities of active ingredient in a homoeopathic remedy mean that they can easily lose their potency. This is called antidoting. It is extremely important therefore, to store and take them in the correct manner to avoid antidoting the remedy. This should be explained to patients when counter-prescribing homoeopathic remedies.

Administration

The remedy should not be handled because impurities and sweat on the hands may reduce the homoeopathic potency. It should be transferred to the mouth on a clean metal spoon or via the lid of its container. As remedies are absorbed through the oral mucosa, they should be sucked or chewed or allowed to dissolve in the mouth - not swallowed.

The remedies should not be taken when there is any strong flavour in the mouth which could interfere with the homoeopathic potency - for example curry, coffee, toothpaste, mint, tobacco or any conventional drugs. The mouth can be cleaned by rinsing with water, and most practitioners advise taking the remedy around 15-30 minutes before or after eating, drinking, smoking or cleaning teeth.

Storage

Homoeopathic remedies should be stored in their original container, away from sunlight and strongly-smelling substances such as perfumes, aromatherapy oils, disinfectants, mothballs and menthol inhalants.

Side effects

Due to the extreme dilutions involved, there are no known side effects or contraindications to homoeopathy. However, because lactose is used in the formulation of homoeopathic tablets, granules and pillules, patients with lactose intolerance should seek advice from their homoeopath or a doctor if their symptoms are persistent or deteriorate.

Interactions

There are no known interactions between homoeopathic remedies and other medicines, so it is acceptable to recommend a homoeopathic remedy alongside a conventional treatment.

Summary of advice on handling remedies

• Do not touch the remedy
• Suck or chew the remedy
• Do not take the remedy when there is any strong flavour in the mouth
• Store the remedy in its original container, away from sunlight and strongly-smelling substances

As with everything, practice and familiarity are key. The better you get to know the remedies and their reactions the more accurate your selection will be and therefore the more effective the remedies will become.

INDEX OF SYMPTOMS AND GUIDE TO SELECTING HOMOEOPATHIC REMEDIES

1. Note down your main symptoms and any strong likes and dislikes that may arise from your symptoms.

2. Study the 'index of symptoms' following.

3. Carefully look at the 'medicines and their indications' (pages 27–35) and select the medicine that most closely matches your symptoms.

Remember that when selecting a remedy you do not always have to experience all the symptoms listed nor do you have to exhibit all the likes and dislikes - these are often expressed as an extreme which may not always apply. Simply try to match up with the set of symptoms most similar to yours.

Under each ailment and condition a number of remedies are listed alphabetically. Sometimes other homoeopathic remedies might also be more appropriate and effective but those suggested are the ones that are most widely available.

This guide to self-treatment relates to ailments that can be treated in the home environment. If you are suffering from a chronic condition, or where the symptoms are serious or prolonged you should always consult a doctor or a qualified homoeopath first.

SYMPTOM	DESCRIPTION	REMEDY
Abdomen painful	Where food lies like a stone in the stomach, feels better after resting	*Bryonia*
	Bloated after a light meal, much flatulence	*Lycopodium*
	Flatulence and colic, after eating or drinking alcohol	*Nux vom*
Abscesses	Patient susceptible to skin infections. Parts tense and painful	*Hepar sulph*
	Tense and painful	*Hypericum*
	Mouth abscesses	*Merc sol*
	When infected fluid has been released but is slow to clear	*Silicea*
Acidity	From nervous anticipation of coming events	*Argent nit*
	Severe heartburn, after only a little food, worse from cold food and drink and around 4–8 pm	*Lycopodium*

14

SYMPTOM	DESCRIPTION	REMEDY
Acne	In those with a ruddy complexion	*Belladonna*
	Where there are many pustules	*Hepar sulph*
	In those with fair complexion	*Pulsatilla*
	Where there is scarring	*Silicea*
	In cases resistant to treatment	*Sulphur*
Adenoids	Enlarged	*Calc phos*
Appetite, excessive	Feeling of emptiness even after a meal	*Cal. carb*
	Even at night, but is easily satisfied	*Lycopodium*
Appetite, loss of	Aversion to food. Hunger in the evening prevents sleep	*Ignatia*
	Continual craving, with loss of appetite	*Arsen alb*
Arthritis	Where there is redness and much swelling	*Apis mel*
	If the joints are bruised	*Arnica*
	When there is no relief from pain	*Bryonia*
	Where bone is affected	*Calc fluor*
	Pains are variable and go from joint to joint	*Pulsatilla*
Bad breath	Bitter taste in the mouth on waking	*Kali phos*
	Metallic taste in the mouth	*Merc sol*
Bereavement	Where the death is sudden and the shock severe	*Aconite*
	Prolonged mourning. Cannot get over the loss of a loved one	*Ignatia*
Bilious attack	Where food lies like a stone in the stomach	*Bryonia*
	Sour taste and nausea after eating, especially after over-eating	*Nux vom*
Bites, animal	For initial treatment However patients should always seek medical attention	*Aconite*
Body odour	Profuse, sour, sticky sweat, day and night, with skin very sensitive to the touch	*Hepar sulph*
	Perspiration which stains the clothes yellow	*Merc sol*
	Profuse sweat at night, chest, back, and thighs. Sweats while seated	*Sepia*
	Where injuries tend to suppurate	*Silicea*
	Where there is unhealthy-looking skin and where feet are particularly a problem	*Sulphur*
	Sweating only on uncovered parts, covered parts are dry	*Thuja*

SYMPTOM	DESCRIPTION	REMEDY
Boils	When there is much redness and heat	Belladonna
	When little injuries turn septic, develop into boils and are intolerably painful. The patient is chilly, the boil is hot	Hepar sulph
	When every little injury tends to become infected. The patient is chilly, the boil is cold	Silicea
Bone injuries	To promote healing particularly where fracture is slow to heal	Calc phos
	Recovery from all kinds of bone injuries is aided with	Nux vom
	Suitable for all musculo-skeletal strains or sprains	Ruta grav
Brain fatigue	Nervous breakdown, trembling of the body, worse from alcohol	Argent nit
	Mental exhaustion, dull, sluggish. Excitement causes diarrhoea	Gelsemium
	Due to excess mental effort	Kali phos
	Due to a dread of having to make any mental effort	Silicea
Bronchitis	Rattling of mucous in the bronchial tubes	Ipecac
Bruises	Fundamental for all bruising whatever the cause	Arnica
	If skin is broken apply a thin smear of Calendula ointment	
Bunions	Throbbing, red, hot, swollen joint. Worse from pressure or movement	Belladonna
	Very stiff, swollen joint with shooting pain. Worse after rest and improves with movement	Rhus tox
	See chiropodist	
Carbuncle	When extremely painful to touch and cannot bear contact of the dressing	Hepar sulph
	To help reduce infection	Silicea
Catarrh	Head colds with thick yellow green discharge	Calc fluor
	Colds with watering eyes and streaming nose	Euphrasia
	Thick yellow-green discharge	Pulsatilla
	Stringy discharge	Kali bich
Change of life	In fair blue-eyed women	Pulsatilla
	In dark-haired women	Sepia
Chestiness	Dry painful cough	Bryonia
	For those who catch colds easily which go onto the chest	Sulphur

SYMPTOM	DESCRIPTION	REMEDY
Chilblains	Intolerably itchy, swollen and stinging pain	Apis mel
	Itching, burning, bluish-red, and swollen. Unbearable in the heat of the bed	Pulsatilla
	Burning, itching, aching – often with muscle weakness. Worse after cold, wet, weather	Rhus tox
	Cracked, chapped skin with burning pain	Calc carb
	Intense burning and uncontrollable itching	Sulphur
	For external use	
Chilliness	For those who always hug the fire or radiator	Arsen alb
	For those with cold hands	Calc carb
	When the chilliness is intense	Hepar sulph
	Especially in the evening	Sepia
Colds	Sudden onset after exposure to draughts and cold winds	Aconite
	Symptoms are influenza-like	Gelsemium
	Much sneezing. Runny nose	Nat mur
Colic	Where there is flatulence	Argent nit
	Better when 'doubled up'	Belladonna
	Better when lying still	Bryonia
Concentration	Cannot concentrate	Apis mel
Confusion	Acute/sudden onset. Patient restless and afraid	Belladonna
	Confusion often associated with senile dementia	Lycopodium
Conjunctivitis	Thick, copious discharge. Sticky eyes in morning, eyes feel swollen	Argent nit
	Extremely sensitive to light. Pain extending behind eyeballs, vision sometimes blurred	Hepar sulph
Constipation	Ineffectual urging	Nax vom
	Stool recedes when partly expelled	Silicea
	Large painful stools	Sulphur
Coughs	Dry painful cough	Bryonia
	Rattling chesty cough associated with infection	Hepar sulph
	Sudden onset of a wheezy, chesty cough	Ipecac
	Ticklish, dry cough, feverish and chilly	Nux vom
	Chesty cough in day with yellow/green phlegm. Changes to dry cough at night. Worse in hot stuffy room	Pulsatilla

SYMPTOM	DESCRIPTION	REMEDY
Cramp	In calf muscles	*Arsen alb*
	Night cramps common, mainly in calf muscles	*Calc carb*
	Cramps due to exercise or occupational activity	*Gelsemium*
Croup	Spasmodic cough	*Calc fluor*
	Occurs after midnight	*Hepar sulph*
	Brought on by fright	*Ignatia*
Cuts	Use a natural healing ointment in conjunction with	*Hypericum*
Cystitis	Stinging pains when passing water	*Apis mel*
	High temperature	*Belladonna*
	Where there are pink deposits in the urine	*Lycopodium*
	When easily distressed by condition	*Pulsatilla*
Dandruff	Where there is scaling of the scalp	*Graphites*
	Moist dandruff	*Sepia*
Dentist, visit to	To reduce pain after teeth extractions and to promote healing	*Arnica*
	Useful for bruising and healing after dental surgery	*Hypericum*
Depression	In emotional individuals and bereavement	*Ignatia*
	Especially women who are easily depressed	*Sepia*
Diarrhoea	Brought on by excitement and worry about coming events	*Argent nit*
	Brought on by mild food poisoning	*Arsen alb*
	Chronic, yellow, offensive, urgent stool, driving patient out of bed in the morning	*Sulphur*
Dyspepsia	Due to nervous excitement about coming events	*Argent nit*
	Much flatulence, in chilly persons, who like fresh air	*Carbo veg*
	Heartburn after only a little food, with colic pains, often around 4–8 pm	*Lycopodium*
Earache	Where there is redness, heat and throbbing	*Belladonna*
	Where there is discharge from the ears	*Graphites*
	Worse at night, with smelly, yellow discharge	*Merc sol*
Eczema	Skin cracked and weeping	*Graphites*
	Very sensitive to touch	*Hepar Sulph*
	At the borders of the hair	*Nat mur*
	Much itching, uncontrollable desire to scratch, results in burning and smarting	*Sulphur*

18

SYMPTOM	DESCRIPTION	REMEDY
Exhaustion	Following physical effort	*Arnica*
	After diarrhoea or sickness	*Arsen alb*
	After mental effort	*Kali phos*
Eyes, inflamed, burning, watering	Unable to bear bright light	*Euphrasia*
Eyelids, swollen	Particularly lower eyelids	*Apis mel*
Face flushed	Red, hot, burning	*Belladonna*
Fat, excess	Excessive appetite	*Calc carb*
	Accompanied by unhealthy skin	*Graphites*
	In shy and emotional individuals	*Pulsatilla*
Fear	Following a frightening incident. Rapid breathing and palpitations, restless and irritable	*Aconite*
	Extremely negative always expecting the worst at every opportunity. Great fear to the point of terror	*Arsen alb*
Fear of coming events	Especially when appearing before an audience	*Argent nit*
	Fear of new situations, anxious before any performance related event. Nervous, sweats under stress	*Lycopodium*
	A sense of failure. 'Examination nerves'	*Gelsemium*
Flatulence	Due to eating sweets, cheese, fats and salty foods	*Argent nit*
	Brings up large amount of wind	*Carbo veg*
Fractures	Where they are slow to heal	*Calc phos*
	General medicine for fractures, dislocations and bone injuries	*Ruta grav*
Giddiness	When looking up at a height or looking down from a height, and when over water, or from mental exertion	*Argent nit*
	Due to exhaustion and weakness	*Kali phos*
Gout	With a fear of being touched	*Arnica*
	Painful inflammation of joints of the fingers	*Calc fluor*
	Painful joints, considerable pain	*Lycopodium*
Gums	Swollen	*Apis mel*
	Gum-boil	*Calc fluor*
	Inflamed and pyorrhoea	*Calc phos*
	Ulcers	*Merc sol*
Haemorrhoids	See PILES	

SYMPTOM	DESCRIPTION	REMEDY
Hay fever	Burning, watering eyes	*Euphrasia*
	Symptoms better in the open air	*Pulsatilla*
	In chilly individuals, often worse on waking	*Silicea*
Headache	Painful, watering eyes and unable to bear bright light	*Euphrasia*
	Pain lessened by bending head backwards	*Hypericum*
	Humming in the ears	*Kali phos*
	Hammering headache preceded by misty vision or zig-zag lights	*Nat mur*
Heartburn	Accompanied by stomach pain	*Calc phos*
	Often from over eating and drinking, or stress related	*Nux vom*
	For recurrent heartburn. Much flatulence and sour taste in mouth	*Sulphur*
Hiccups	After food, especially if eaten too quickly. Heartburn and flatulence	*Lycopodium*
Hoarseness	Following cold, damp weather	*Carbo veg.*
Horse-fly bites	To help reduce swelling	*Hypericum*
Hot flushes	Face red and flushed	*Graphites*
	Useful for menopausal women. Profuse sweating. Joints inflamed	*Sepia*
Housemaid's knee	Where there is much inflammation	*Nat mur*
Hunger, excessive	Even at night, but is easily satisfied	*Lycopodium*
Incontinence	Stinging and burning	*Apis mel*
	Where there is liking for salty food	*Nat mur*
Indigestion	Accompanied by much flatulence	*Carbo veg*
	Due to nervous causes	*Kali Phos*
	Due to over-eating	*Nux vom*
Insomnia	Much twisting and turning	*Aconite*
	Over-tiredness, bed feels hard	*Arnica*
	Jerks on going to sleep, often with nightmares	*Belladonna*
	Sweating of the head during sleep	*Calc Carb*
	Frequent yawning but can't sleep	*Ignatia*
	Limbs hot and must be placed outside bedclothes. Requires extra pillow	*Sulphur*

20

SYMPTOM	DESCRIPTION	REMEDY
Irritability	From jealousy, fright, anger or grief	*Apis mel*
	Much twisting and turning	*Aconite*
	Impulsiveness, always rushed. Motivated by a fear of failure	*Argent Nit*
	Very ill-tempered and easily aggravated	*Bryonia*
Itching	Itching scalp	*Argent nit*
	Skin, worse on getting warm	*Merc sol*
	Scratching pleasurable, but results in burning	*Sulphur*
Joints	Swollen	*Belladonna*
	Painful and rheumatic	*Rhus tox*
Laryngitis	Loss of voice/hoarseness which persists for no apparent reason	*Argent nit*
	Irritating sore throat with fish bone sensation. Pain rotates to ears. Chesty cough	*Hepar sulph*
Ligaments, painful	Due to over-exertion	*Rhus tox*
Light, intolerance to	Watery, stinging eyes	*Euphrasia*
Lips, dry	Excessive thirst	*Bryonia*
Listless	And unsettled	*Apis mel*
Liverishness	In early morning	*Nux vom*
Lumbago	Very deep-seated	*Calc fluor*
	Much restlessness	*Rhus tox*
Menstrual pain	Tenderness of the breasts	*Calc carb*
	Accompanied with a headache	*Calc phos*
	Accompanied with depression	*Lycopodium*
	When both sad and irritable	*Nat mur*
	Tearful with painful breasts	*Pulsatilla*
Mental strain	Due to overwork and worry about the future	*Argent nit*
Migraine	Preceded by misty vision or zig-zag lights	*Nat nur*
	Beginning in the neck, coming over the head, and ending in one eye	*Silicea*
	Blurred vision before headache	*Kali Bich*
Milk, aversion	Where there is a craving for eggs and sweets	*Calc Carb*

21

SYMPTOM	DESCRIPTION	REMEDY
Mouth, taste in	Sweetish, metallic taste, saliva coppery	*Merc sol*
	Ulcers	*Merc sol*
Muscular soreness	After exposure to cold. Particularly for muscle pain in back and limbs	*Bryonia*
	After prolonged exercise	*Arnica*
Nausea	Burning pains in abdomen and heartburn	*Arsen alb*
	Sudden onset of nausea and sickness where vomiting brings no relief	*Ipecac*
	Useful for vomiting after drinking alcohol	*Kali bich*
	Induced by over-eating, over-drinking or stress	*Nux vom*
'Nerves'	Due to worry about coming events	*Argent nit*
	Unable to cope with life	*Gelsemium*
	Extremely irritable with digestive problems	*Nux vom*
Neuralgia	Acute onset. Red, hot face with dry skin. Pain tends to be left-sided	*Aconite*
	Right-sided pain with twitching muscles. Violent pains come and go rapidly. Flushed hot, burning face	*Belladonna*
Nose	Caused by injury, patient may be shocked. Nose feels bruised and tender	*Arnica*
	Running, with influenza-like symptoms	*Gelsemium*
	Severe nosebleed with hot blood and red face	*Belladonna*
	Nose runs like a tap	*Nat mur*
Overweight	Enlarged glands	*Calc carb*
	Tendency to skin ailments	*Graphites*
Overwork, effects from	When long hours have been worked with much mental strain	*Argent nit*
	When there is nervous exhaustion	*Kali phos*
Pains, burning	As a result of insect stings	*Apis mel*
	Feet burn in the bed. Burning, itching piles	*Sulphur*
Pains, shooting	Very sharp shooting pains which may come and go. Areas sore and tender	*Hypericum*
Periods, irregularities with	See also Menstrual Pain	
	Periods are too early and may be excessive	*Calc phos*
	In fair-haired, blue-eyed women. Periods are delayed, scanty, yet protracted	*Pulsatilla*
	In dark-haired women. Periods delayed	*Sepia*

22

SYMPTOM	DESCRIPTION	REMEDY
Piles	Bleeding, protruding and itching piles	*Calc fluor*
	Where there is a prolapse of the rectum	*Ruta grav*
	Sensitive piles	*Hypericum*
	Protruding piles with itching pains	*Ignatia*
	Itching piles	*Nux vom*
Premenstrual tension	Breasts swollen and painful. Tired and lacking in energy	*Calc carb*
	Increase in weight	*Graphites*
	Depressed and irritable. Symptoms disappear as soon as period starts	*Lycopodium*
	Irritable, sad, moody. Lower back pain	*Nat mur*
	Quarrelsome	*Nux vom*
	Periods irregular. Breasts swollen, painful. Over-sensitive and moved to tears easily	*Pulsatilla*
	Sad, apathetic, great exhaustion during period	*Sepia*
Psoriasis	In intelligent, tidy individuals	*Arsen alb*
	In cautious, indecisive individuals	*Graphites*
	In over-sensitive individuals given to quick, hasty speech	*Hepa sulph*
	In deep-thinking, independent individuals	*Sulphur*
Restlessness	In those with acute imagination	*Aconite*
	Due to debility and exhaustion	*Arsen alb*
	Great apprehension at night	*Rhus tox*
Rheumatism	In back and limbs	*Apis mel*
	Fear of being touched	*Arnica*
	Greatly aggravated by movement	*Bryonia*
	Use after Rhus tox.	*Calc carb*
	Worse on beginning to move, but improves with continued gentle movement	*Rhus tox*
	Pain in tendons and muscles	*Ruta grav*
School phobia	In sensitive children	*Gelsemium*
Sciatica	Made worse in cold, damp weather and at night. Searing pains which improve on movement	*Rhus tox*
Shingles	Where the scalp is affected	*Rhus tox*
Shivering	But prefers the window to be open	*Carbo veg*

SYMPTOM	DESCRIPTION	REMEDY
Sickness	Burning pains in the stomach	*Arsen alb*
	Air sickness	*Belladonna*
	Where there is nausea	*Ipecac*
	Sickness and vomiting after drinking alcohol	*Kali bich*
	Caused by over-eating	*Nux vom*
Sinus affections	Catarrh with stringy discharge	*Kali bich*
	Tearing pain in head, from root of nose extending to forehead with nausea	*Nat mur*
	Pain begins at the back of the head and settles over the eyes	*Silicea*
Skin disorders	Irregular blotches	*Argent nit*
	Cracked, weeping eczema	*Graphites*
	Better for scratching	*Calc carb*
	Injuries tend to become infected	*Hepar Sulph*
	Itchy skin which feels worse on getting warm	*Merc sol*
	Itching skin, scratching relieves, but results in burning	*Sulphur*
Sprains	Where there is bruising	*Arnica*
	Sprains of joints or tendons	*Rhus tox*
	Sprains of wrists or ankles	*Ruta grav*
Splinter, sensation of	At the back of the throat	*Hepar Sulph*
Stings (Insect)	Painful, bright red and swollen	*Apis mel*
	Bee or wasp, painful to touch, and bruised	*Arnica*
Stomach, upset	Where there is sickness and burning pains	*Arsen alb*
Stomach, painful to touch	When food lies like a stone in the stomach	*Bryonia*
Styes	Sticky discharge	*Graphites*
	At onset take	*Pulsatilla*
	And warts	*Thuja*
Sunburn	Redness, heat and burning. Sometimes swollen and throbbing area	*Belladonna*
Suppuration	Cracked skin	*Graphites*
	When there is great sensitivity to the slightest touch	*Hepar sulph*
Swallowing difficulty in	Sore throat and runny nose	*Gelsemium*

24

SYMPTOM	DESCRIPTION	REMEDY
Synovitis	Associated with sprains	*Ruta grav*
Tendons	Painful from over-exertion	*Rhus tox*
	Painful from rheumatism	*Ruta grav*
Thirst, absence of	Accompanied with a swollen throat	*Apis mel*
	Even with a high temperature	*Gelsemium*
	Even though the mouth may be dry	*Pulsatilla*
Thirst	High temperature	*Aconite*
	For cold drinks	*Bryonia*
	Due to the over-use of salt	*Nat mur*
	Mouth feels dry. There is a desire for milk	*Rhus tox*
Throat, sore	Following exposure to dry winds	*Aconite*
	Dry and burning	*Arsen alb*
	Excess of saliva	*Merc sol*
Thrush (mouth)	Much mouth watering	*Merc sol*
	Where the lips are affected	*Nat mur*
Tinnitus	Accompanied by vertigo and nausea	*Carbo veg*
	Where catarrh makes worse	*Pulsatilla*
	When noises are worse at night	*Sulphur*
Tiredness	Following physical effort	*Arnica*
	After diarrhoea or sickness	*Arsen alb*
	After mental effort	*Kali phos*
Tonsilitis	Much inflammation	*Hepar sulph*
Toothache	Worse for cold air and drinks	*Calc carb*
	In poor teeth	*Calc fluor*
	Worse from hot and cold, but better when cheek is rubbed	*Merc sol*
'Touchiness'	As a result of fussing	*Hepar sulph*
Travel sickness	Accompanied by restlessness and fear	*Aconite*
	Great sensitivity to least movement	*Nux vom*
	The need to vomit	*Ipecac*
	Air sickness	*Belladonna*
Urticaria	Burning and stinging. Worse in heat, better for cold bathing	*Apis mel*
	After strenuous exercise or stress	*Nat mur*
	Accompanied by indigestion	*Ruta grav*

SYMPTOM	DESCRIPTION	REMEDY
Varicose veins	Usually brought on by prolonged periods of standing. Painful, uncomfortable, restless legs	*Aconite*
	Accompanied by poor circulation	*Carbo veg*
	Medical advice should always be taken	
Vertigo	Where there is buzzing in the ears	*Argent nit*
	Worse when turning in bed	*Belladonna*
	With vomiting	*Bryonia*
	Worse when looking up	*Calc carb*
	Where there is nausea and tinnitus	*Carbo veg*
	Accompanied by trembling	*Gelsemium*
	Accompanied by a headache	*Nat mur*
	Accompanied by nausea	*Nux vom*
Voice, loss of	Hoarseness	*Carbo veg*
	Due to over-use of the voice	*Kali phos*
Vomiting	See SICKNESS	
Warts	Use a suitable external application and take	*Thuja*
Washday hands	From constant immersion in water	*Sepia*
Whitlow	Inflammation, heat, throbbing and tenderness	*Belladonna*
	Accompanied by marked whiteness of skin	*Calc fluor*
	Throbbing, infected, worse at night	*Hepar sulph*
	When infection is slow to develop	*Silicea*
Wounds, lacerated or punctured	Where nerve endings have been affected; pain travelling upwards. Suitable for horse-fly bites.	*Hypericum*

THE MEDICINES AND THEIR INDICATIONS

MEDICINE/AILMENT OR CONDITION	REMARKS

1. Aconite (Aconitum napellus)

Symptoms are sudden, violent and brief
Exposure to draughts or a cold wind
Dry suffocating cough
Sore throat following exposure to cold dry winds
High temperature with great thirst
Great pain
Bereavement
Animal bites
Travel sickness
Anxiety, restlessness, fear, grief
Insomnia

Worse:
at midnight. When lying on affected side, in a warm room, in tobacco smoke, in cold winds, listening to music

Better:
in the open air, with bedclothes thrown off

2. Apis mel. (Apis mellifica)

Effects of insect stings
Burning stinging pains
Cystitis
Swelling of lower eyelids
Absence of thirst
Arthritis
Rheumatism
Listless
Cannot concentrate
Swollen gums
Incontinence
Urticaria

Apis mel. is indicated in cases where irritability and despondency result from fright, jealousy, anger or grief

Worse:
during late afternoon, after sleeping, from heat, when touched, in closed and heated rooms

Better:
in open air, from cold bathing

3. Argent. nit. (Argentum nitricum)

Acidity, dyspepsia
Craving for sweet food, cheese, fats or salt followed by upset stomach with much flatulence
Colic
Headache
Dizziness from overwork and mental strain
Vertigo with overwork in the ears
Conjunctivitis
Itching scalp
Irregular blotches on skin

Suited to impulsive, irritable or nervous people who tend to worry about the uncertainties of the future Helpful when taken before a difficult undertaking (e.g. making a speech)

Worse:
in warmth, after eating sweet foods, from overwork, with worry about the future

4. Arnica (Arnica montana)

Use after any injury
Bruises
Sprains
Physical exhaustion following sustained exercise, e.g. a day's gardening or a long walk
Insomnia due to over-tiredness

Worse:
from touch, from motion, in damp, cold conditions

Better:
when lying down, with head low

MEDICINE/AILMENT OR CONDITION   REMARKS

Arnica (contd)
Muscles ache all over
Bed feels too hard – constant desire to
move to a soft part
Cannot bear to be touched
Great sensitivity to pain
Gout, rheumatism with a fear of being touched

5. *Arsen. alb. (Arsenicum album)*
Restlessness
Anxiety and fear
Burning pains
Throat dry and burning
Burning pain in the stomach
Thirst with the desire to sip little and often
Food poisoning
Cramps in calves
Cannot bear the sight or smell of food
Psoriasis

Suited to excessively tidy,
intelligent and precise
individuals

Worse:
after midnight, between 1 and
2 pm, at the coast, from cold and
wet weather, after eating ice
cream or cold drinks, when
feeling hot

Better:
by keeping warm, with cool
air round the head

6. *Belladonna (tropa belladonna)*
Brightly flushed face
Swollen joints
Insomnia
Vertigo
Facial neuralgia
Severe throbbing earache
Throbbing headache
Dry hacking cough
Air sickness
Acne
Cystitis
Whitlow
Colic

Suited to lively cheerful
individuals

Worse:
in the afternoon and at night,
from noise, from touch,
when lying down

Better:
from warmth, while sitting erect

7. *Bryonia (Bryonia alba)*
Irritability
Chestiness – colds often go down into the chest
Dryness
Dry painful cough, often violent
Dry lips
Thirst, especially for cold drinks
Food lies like a stone in the stomach
which is too painful to touch
Sits with knees up
Colic
Diarrhoea after eating over-ripe fruit
Arthritis
Vertigo

Worse:
from any movement, from warmth

Better:
from cold, from cold food and
drinks, from pressure (except on
the abdomen), from rest,
while lying on the painful side

MEDICINE/AILMENT OR CONDITION	REMARKS

8. Calc. carb. (Calcarea carbonica)

Excessive appetite	Suited to quiet, shy, sensitive
Overweight	people who are subject to
Dislikes milk	depression. Often a feeling of
Craving for eggs and sweets	being looked at by everyone and
May feel generally better when constipated	a fear of being laughed at.
Tendency to feel the cold and to catch	Embarrassment when entering a
cold easily	room full of strangers.
Cold hands	
Cracked skin in the winter	*Worse:*
Itching skin	from cold, in damp weather,
Profuse periods	at night, from standing
Period pains	
Premenstrual tension	*Better:*
Toothache	in dry weather, from warmth
Vertigo	(avoid sun), while lying on the
Insomnia, with much sweating once asleep	painful side
Use after Rhus tox, for rheumatism	

9. Calc. fluor. (Calcarea fluorica)

Head colds with thick greenish-yellow discharge	*Worse:*
Catarrh	after rest, from damp weather
Cough with tiny lumps of tough mucus	
Croup	*Better:*
Piles – bleeding, protruding, itching	after a little movement,
Varicose veins	from warm applications
Whitlow	
Gum-boil	
Toothache	
Arthritis	

10. Carbo veg. (Carbo vegetabilis)

Indigestion with excessive flatulence	*Worse:*
Mild food poisoning after eating fish	after eating fatty foods
Ailments following cold damp weather	during warm damp weather
Shivering but likes open window	in the evening and at night
Cold limbs at night	
Hoarseness	*Better:*
Loss of voice	on bringing up wind, from cold
Tinnitus with nausea and vertigo	

11. Euphrasia (Euphrasia officinalis)

Cold with watering eyes and streaming nose	*Worse:*
Inflamed eyes which sting and burn	in the evening, in bed,
Conjunctivitis	when indoors, from warmth,
Inability to bear bright light	in bright light
Hayfever	
	Better:
	in dim light or darkness,
	from cold applications

29

MEDICINE/AILMENT OR CONDITION	REMARKS
12. Gelsemium sempervirens)	
Influenza	Suited to excitable people who
Sneezing	suffer from 'nerves', have great
Sore throat	difficulty in coping with life's
Symptoms of flushing, aching, trembling	problems and by whom even
'Tight' headache	the simplest tasks are anticipated
Heavy eyes	with nervousness and worry
Shivering	
Weary with heavy, aching muscles	*Worse:*
Absence of thirst even with high temperature	about 10 am, in hot rooms,
Difficulty in swallowing	when exposed to the sun,
Running nose	before thunderstorms,
Vertigo	on receiving bad news
School phobia	
	Better:
	in the open air, after passing water
13. Graphites (Graphites)	
Unhealthy skin	Suited to individuals who are by
Eczema	nature extremely cautious and who
Tendency for injuries to become infected	find difficulty in making decisions
Cracked finger tips	
Overweight	*Worse:*
Constipation	at night, during and after periods,
Tinnitus	in draughts
Earache	
Sinus trouble	*Better:*
Styes	in the dark, from wrapping up
Dandruff	
Hot flushes	
Premenstrual tension	
14. Hepar sulph. (Hepar sulphuris)	
Skin highly sensitive to touch (even clothing	Suited to acutely sensitive
on affected parts is very painful)	individuals of fair hair and
Injuries tend to become infected	complexion, who speak quickly,
Eczema	dislike fuss and prefer to be
Acne	left alone
Crack in the middle of the lower lip	
Whitlow	*Worse:*
Intense chilliness	in cold air, when lying on the
Croup	painful side, when affected parts
Cough brought on by the least exposure	are touched
to the cold air	
Wheezing	*Better:*
Sensation of a splinter at the back of the throat	from warmth, from wrapping up
Earache	(especially the head),
Tonsilitis	in damp wet weather

MEDICINE/AILMENT OR CONDITION   REMARKS

15. *Hypericum (Hypericum perforatum)*
Very painful cuts and wounds
Lacerated wounds involving nerve endings
Falls injuring spine, especially coccyx
Headache with a floating sensation as a
result of a fall
Blows on fingers or toes, torn nail
Horse-fly bites
Sensitive, bleeding piles
Abscess, tense and painful

Worse:
from the cold and damp
from touch, in a closed room

Better:
while bending head backwards

16. *Ignatia (Ignatia amara)*
Fright
Prolonged grief
Piles which protrude easily with stitching
pains in the rectum and which are better
while walking
Sore throat relieved by swallowing
Croup
Dislike of tobacco and tobacco smoke
Piercing headache
Insomnia with much yawning

Suited to emotional and
sensitive people who are easily
moved to tears and who prefer
to be left alone

Worse:
cold air, strong odours,
tobacco smoke, coffee, alcohol

Better:
warmth, change of position
while eating

17. *Ipecac, (Ipecacuanha)*
Any illness where there is nausea and sickness
Travel sickness, no relief from vomiting
Bronchitis
Rattling of mucus in the bronchial tubes
with nausea and sickness

Worse:
in winter and dry weather,
in a warm room

Better:
in open air, resting with eyes closed

18. *Kali. bich. (Kalium bichromicum)*
Complaints brought on by a change to
hot weather
Catarrh with a stringy discharge
Sinus troubles
Hard cough with stringy sputum or in plugs
Sore throat
Migraine – blurred vision before headache
Pains move rapidly from place to place
Nausea and vomiting after alcohol

Worse:
in the morning, from alcohol,
especially beer, during hot weather

Better:
from heat

19. *Kali. phos. (Kalium phosphoricum)*
Mental tiredness from overwork
Nervous exhaustion
Nervous indigestion
Indigestion following a 'working lunch'
Exhaustion following long periods of preparation
for examinations

Worse:
from noise, excitement, worry
from mental and physical exertion

Better:
during gentle movement

31

MEDICINE/AILMENT OR CONDITION   REMARKS

Kali. phos. *(cont)*
mental effort
Loss of voice or hoarseness after over-exertion
and constant use of the voice
Giddiness from exhaustion and weakness
Dry tongue in the morning

20. Lycopodium (Lycopodium clavatum)

Irritability	Suited to people who are intense,
Dislike of exercise	conscientious and of keen
Fear of failure	intellect but who nevertheless
Preference to be alone (but with somebody near)	feel insecure. They cannot endure
Excessive hunger even at night but which is	contradiction but seek argument
easily satisfied	May be irritable, especially in the
Craving for sweet foods even though they	morning. Symptoms (mostly on
cause indigestion	the right side)
Coldness in one foot (usually the right)	
while the other is warm	*Worse:*
Pains which go from right to left	between 4 and 8 pm, in stuffy
Dislike of cold weather but the better for it	rooms, from cold air, food, liquid
Cystitis	sensitive to music, loud and
Period pain	sudden noise
Premenstrual tension	
Gout	*Worse:*
Hiccough with acidity	after warm drinks, food,
	on loosening clothing
	in fresh air, activity

21. Merc. sol. (Mercurius solubilis)

Feverish head cold (with weakness and trembling)	*Worse:*
Sore throat with excessive saliva	at night, in a warm room,
Tongue flabby and indented	in bed, lying on right side,
Metallic taste in mouth	during wet or changeable
Mouth ulcers	weather, and the least draught
Thrush (mouth)	
Thirst	*Better:*
Toothache, earache	at rest, after rising or sitting up,
Abscesses	at high altitudes
Chilliness at onset of a cold	
Diarrhoea with straining	
itching skin	

22. Nat. mur. (Natrum muriaticum)

Sneezy colds	Suited to those of a pale
Nose runs like a tap (treat quickly at the onset)	complexion and oily skin who
Sinus	tend to feel insecure, worry about
Eczema	the future and are easily moved
Thrush (mouth)	to tears. They are irritable and
Urticaria	quarrelsome, do not wish to be
Incontinence	ignored but dislike consolation
Vertigo	

32

MEDICINE/AILMENT OR CONDITION

REMARKS

Nat. mur. (cont)
Menstrual pain when both sad and irritable
Premenstrual tension
Migraine
Housemaid's knee
Thirst
Dislike of bread
Use of much salt on food
Exhaustion

Worse:
in mid-morning, at the seaside,
although can be the reverse
lying down, stress

Better:
in the open air, bright days, while
lying on the right side, washing in
cold water after sweating

23. Nux vom. (Nux vomica)
'Nerves'
Nervous indigestion
Over-sensitive to noise, odours, light, music
Trifling ailments unbearable
Ill effects of over-eating or drinking
Early morning liverishness
Travel sickness
Fussiness about food, liking for fatty foods
Indigestion
Dislike of coffee and tobacco smoke
Pain, like a stone in the stomach, two to
three hours after eating
Constipation with ineffectual urging
Itching piles
Stuffy colds
Raw throat
Vertigo
Premenstrual tension

Suited to thin, dark people who
are inclined to be impatient
and irritable

Worse:
between 3 and 4 pm, from cold,
dry weather and draught

Better:
in the evening, from being
covered, at rest, from warmth,
after waking in the morning

24. Pulsatilla (Pulsatilla nigricans)
Catarrh (yellow-green thick discharge)
Hayfever
Styes (especially on upper lids)
Change of life
Menstrual pain
Premenstrual tension
Periods scanty yet protracted
Cystitis
Acne
Tinnitus
Arthritis
Rapid change in symptoms – from feeling well
to feeling miserable
Pains shift rapidly
Aversion to fat or greasy food
Absence of thirst (even in fever) though the
mouth may be dry

Suited to persons with fair hair,
blue eyes and fair or pale
complexion (often with pink
patches). They are affectionate,
easily moved to laughter or tears,
shy, never obstinate but like and
seek sympathy. They are sensitive
to reprimand and tend to put on
fat easily. They dislike extremes
of weather

Worse:
in the evening, from heat, after
eating rich foods, from sudden
chilling when hot

Better:
in the open air, from cold
applications, after cold food and
drinks, while lying on the painful

33

MEDICINE/AILMENT OR CONDITION   REMARKS

25. Rhus tox. (Rhus toxicodendron)

Effects of over-exertion, strain operations, etc.
Strains of joints or tendons
Rheumatism, lumbago, sciatica
Pain in ligaments
Shingles
Thirst
Tickling cough
Tongue with red triangular tip
Restlessness

Worse:
on beginning to move*, from cold
and wet, during rest, after midnight

Better:
during warm weather with gentle
movement, from warm applications

*Pain increases on beginning to
move but tends to diminish if a
gentle movement is maintained

26. Ruta grav. (Ruta graveolens)

Injuries to bones – bruised bones,
fractures, dislocations
Sprains of wrists and ankles
Pains as if bruised
Rheumatism with pain in tendons and muscles
Eye strain – eyes burning and aching
Synovitis
Urticaria
Piles with prolapse of the rectum

Worse:
from cold, during wet weather,
while lying down

27. Sepia (Sepia)

Indifference to loved ones
Sadness and fear of being left alone
"All-gone" sensation in the middle of the morning
Sensitive to the cold
Premenstrual tension
Periods suppressed or delayed
Change of life
Hot sweats
Dandruff
Wash-day hands

Suited to people who are easily
depressed, particularly women,
and who are likely to harbour
real or imaginary fears. They have
little interest in work or recreation

Worse:
in the afternoon and evening,
from cold, before thunder,
from tobacco smoke

Better:
in a warm bed, from hot
applications

28. Silicea (Silicea)

Physical and mental debility due to over-
exertion or to over-use of the mind
Boils, carbuncles, abscesses, acne
Bunions
Whitlow
Helps the expulsion of foreign bodies,
e.g. thorns and splinters
Constipation – stool recedes when partly expelled
Migraine
Chronic headache beginning in the neck,
coming over the head and ending in one eye

Suited to persons of light
complexion, fine skin and pale
face who find mental effort
difficult. They have difficulty
facing up to people and problems
and prefer not to have
responsibility.
Despite a dread of work they
have nevertheless excellent
working ability

MEDICINE/AILMENT OR CONDITION	REMARKS

Silicea *(cont)*
Hayfever
Sinus trouble

Worse:
from cold, from being uncovered,
in cold weather, in approaching
winter

Better:
when wrapped up, lying down,
in summer

29. Sulphur (Sulphur)
Unhealthy looking skin
Tendency to skin diseases
Itching skin – scratching pleasurable but
results in burning
Acne
Burning and itching piles
Tendency to sweat easily
Body odour
Orifices of body red (e.g. lips)
Burning pains
Feet must be placed outside bedclothes to cool
Insomnia
Tinnitus
Mid-morning hunger
Large appetite for highly seasoned, spicy
and fatty foods
Liking for sweets
Aggravation from milk
Diarrhoea – driven from bed in the morning
Constipation with large, painful stools
Lack of energy (regained quickly at the
prospect of pleasurable activity)
Tendency to become exhausted quickly
Tendency to catch cold easily which
often goes into the chest
Bed sores

Suited to deep thinking people
who have a nervous yet
independent nature

Worse:
from cold, from dampness,
at the coast

Better:
from warmth, in fresh air

30. Thuja (Thuja occidentalis)
Warty growths
Styes
Pain, which may be accompanied with the
frequent passing of water
Morning headaches
Inability to take food in the morning

Suited to dark-haired,
dark-skinned people with strong,
sometimes inflexible minds

Worse:
from cold, damp weather
bright, direct sun, heat of bed,
at 3 am and 3 pm

Better:
while drawing up a limb, in cool
air, after sweating, from massage

ESPECIALLY FOR CHILDREN

Aconite

Hot, dry skin. Feverish thirst for cold water.

For those prone to catching colds after getting wet.

Give this medicine in the early stages before this condition becomes well established.

Apis mel

Where the child is tearful and fidgety and where there is retention of urine in nursing infants. Shrill, sudden piercing screams whilst asleep or awake.

Argent nit

Usually agitated and fidgety, with an irresistible desire for sweets and sugar; this causes sickness and vomiting of mouthfuls of liquid and greenish diarrhoea.

Arnica

This is a most useful medicine for dealing with the bumps and bruises of childhood. It is especially helpful if the child is shocked after some little mishap. Arnica cream applied externally is also helpful in clearing up a bruised surface. The medicine can be given before and after visiting the dentist to assist the natural healing process.

Arsen alb

Over-tired and irritable even after minimal exertion. Stomach pains from eating fruit, shellfish and rich / oily foods. Often associated with mild food poisoning. Child feels generally worse around midnight and is restless.

Belladonna

The child suffers a sudden attack of symptoms which usually include hot and red skin with flushed face. The attack is often violent and there may be great excitement with vomiting or a severe headache. Use if the child has been exposed to too much sun.

Bryonia

In contrast to Belladonna, symptoms usually come on gradually. The child may be irritable and dislike being lifted or carried. Hard, dry cough with stitching pains in the chest, made worse by movement. Thirst.

Calc phos

For pale, thin, children. The infant wants to suckle all the time and vomits easily. Headaches at time of puberty.

Chamomilla teething granules

This is the medicine for fractious teething infants, best given in granule form. The child whines and wants many things, but immediately throws them away, and is only pacified with constant petting.

Gelsemium

The remedy for influenza. The symptoms are well-known: shivering with cold which may alternate with heat; aching all over. Diarrhoea from emotional excitement. Examination fear in older children.

Hepar sulph

For over-sensitive children who take offence at the slightest thing. Useful where there are splinter like pains, especially the sensation of a bone stuck in the throat. Unhealthy skin, cuts and grazes tend to become infected.

Hypericum

An excellent remedy which promotes healing and relieves pain. Especially good for trapped fingers. Also useful to take if a child has been bitten or scratched by an animal, however in this instance the child should always be referred to a doctor.

Ipecac

Especially good where there is diarrhoea in infants and where the stools are green and slimy. All complaints are accompanied by nausea and frequent shivering and yawning. The onset of the illness is sudden but progresses rapidly and the child screams continuously. Children who are overweight and pale feel nauseous, vomit and have colic and diarrhoea.

Lycopodium

Child wakes up both cross and angry and is inclined to strike, bite, scratch and kick everyone who approaches. Child painfully wishes to urinate and clasps abdomen. There is a red sand deposit in the nappy and a rash where urine has inflamed the skin. Often the right foot is cold whilst the left foot is of normal temperature.

Merc. sol

A useful remedy for toothache, bad breath, mouth ulcers and where the child complains of a bad taste in the mouth. In the case of toothache the child should always be taken to the dentist.

Nux vom

An excellent remedy to give to children who have over-eaten and indulged in rich food. The child will often be irritable and have a sour taste in its mouth, feel nauseous and complain of stomach pains. This may also be followed by a period of constipation where this remedy will also be of help.

Pulsatilla

A good remedy for a child with a mild and gentle disposition who is easily moved to tears. The child may fear the dark and ghosts and like to be fussed over and caressed. It is also a useful remedy for styes.

Rhus tox

A remedy for children who play out in the rain and then complain of having pains the next day. The child often feels better on moving about. These symptoms may also be the result of a visit to a swimming pool.

Silicea

For weak children who eat plenty but whose assimilation is poor. The child is constantly restless, self-willed, touchy and difficult. Often the child is unable to take any form of milk and even the mother's milk causes vomiting and diarrhoea. The child may be chilly even in a warm room and may sweat at night. Sometimes there is bed wetting with a yellow sand deposit in the nappy.

Sulphur

Use when the child is difficult to calm, becomes sulky and will not speak. Warm, hungry babies will kick off their bedcovers. Their lips, eyelids, nostrils and anus are scarlet in colour. The child cannot bear to be washed and its skin may be rough, scaly and itchy.

EXPLANATION OF TERMS IN COMMON USE

Acute: An illness which lasts a short time and with pronounced symptoms.

Aggravation: A temporary worsening of symptoms which may occur during homoeopathic treatment as the remedy brings the infection to the surface whereupon it can be tackled and overcome more easily by the body's natural healing forces.

Allopathy: A word first used by Dr Samuel Hahnemann to describe the ordinary system of medical treatment.

Centesimal: The dilution of one part of substance to ninety-nine parts of diluent. Homoeopathic medicines prepared on this scale are referred to as c or ch.

Chronic: An illness persisting over a long period of time. The symptoms are constantly present or recur frequently.

Classical: Traditional homoeopathy according to the principles established by Dr Samuel Hahnemann.

Constitutional medicine: A medicine prescribed on the basis of character, temperament and general reactions, as well as for the symptoms of the illness.

Decimal: The dilution of one part of substance to nine parts of diluent. Homoeopathic medicines prepared on this scale are referred to as D or x.

Hahnemann: Dr Christian Friedrich Samuel Hahnemann was born in Meissen, 10 April 1755. A brilliant student, Hahnemann read medicine and graduated from the University of Erlangen in 1775. Samuel Hahnemann soon became disillusioned with the medical practices of the time and set about to discover a form of medicine that would be safe, gentle and effective. Through research over a number of years and with the help of friends and followers Hahnemann established the system of Homoeopathic Medicine as it practised today. He died in Paris in 1843 in his late eighties.

Materia medica: A detailed list of homoeopathic remedies, in alphabetical order. These books give the sources of remedies and the symptom picture related to each one. This information is then used to match the symptoms of the patient with those of a medicine.

Medicine pictures: A summary of symptoms that a substance is capable of producing in a healthy person and is therefore appropriate for the treatment of those symptoms.

Modalities: A term applied when the patient feels better or worse. For example heat, lying down, sitting up, fresh air, etc. It is Modalities together with the medicine picture which results in the individual being treated rather than the illness.

Mother tincture: The starting material for the preparation of homoeopathic medicines denoted by the symbol ().

Organon: First published in 1810 and entitled *The Organon of Rational Healing*, this book is considered to be the most important of all Samuel Hahnemann's works, in which he has set out the whole of his philosophy on Homoeopathy.

Polycrests: A medicine of value as a remedy for several conditions or diseases.

Potency: Dr Samuel Hahnemann discovered that the greater the dilution, the more potent the remedy became, therefore a Potency is the strength, or dilution, of a remedy.

Provings: The name given to the systematic testing, by healthy people, of a potential homoeopathic medicine. The purpose of this was to catalogue all the symptoms induced by the substance, experienced by the person taking it. In this way Hahnemann and his followers established many homoeopathic remedies.

Similia similibus currentur: The Law of Similars – 'Let like be treated by like'.

Succussion: Violent shaking, with impact, which takes place at each stage of sequential dilution when preparing a homoeopathic remedy.

Trituration: The method of producing a homoeopathic remedy from a substance which is insoluble. The substance is finely ground and mixed with an appropriate diluent.